Bulletproof Diet Recipes for Frugal & Fast Cooking:

How to Cook Simple and Delicious Weight loss Recipes In No Time And Reclaim Your Energy and Focus

By

By Michele Gilbert

Visit My Amazon Author Page

Table of Contents

Introduction

Are you fed up with the amount of time that you spend in the kitchen? Do you want to save some money and eat healthier? Do you want to lose fat?

Now is the best time to start your weight loss journey and as challenging as it may seem you will be able to reach your goal a lot faster with the proper diet and the proper mindset. This is why I have included some general dieting tips in this eBook.

If you want to save some valuable time and if you want to lose weight you need to bring in a bit of diversity to your diet because you cannot eat the same food every day and expect to have the same results. If you eat the same boring food that people eat in order to lose weight you will end up with a boring diet and this is one of the main cause of failed diets.

After you learn how to use these recipes you will be able to cook your favorite food a lot faster and you will also have plenty of time to use for exercise as if you combine healthy eating with proper exercise you will be able to lose weight very fast.

It is important to keep your daily goals in check and while this may sound a bit intimidating if you are a goal oriented person and if you want to completely change your way of life than you should apply the lessons that you may learn from this eBook because these tips have worked great for me and hopefully they will work great for you as well.

If you are struggling to lose weight and if you feel like you are not achieving the desired results due to poor time management and poor cooking skills you will definitely learn a lot from this book. I used to struggle with losing weight for years and I was also a bad cook. I used to serve a lot of my meals out in town and I have never realized that a slight improvement in my diet can bring such a dramatic change.

If you want to kick start your journey into a healthier lifestyle you will have to completely change your life and you will have to set daily goals. Start your daily goal setting by learning how to cook a different type of healthy meal once/day and keep on learning until you feel like you can cook healthy and delicious food without the aid of a recipe.

If you follow this advice you will be surprised to see that in only two weeks you will be able to cook healthy food on a regular basis. You will start to feel better about yourself and you will also feel healthier. After all, you cannot stay in shape and save money if you eat out all the time.

© Copyright 2015 by Michele Gilbert- All rights reserved.

This document is geared towards providing exact and reliable information in regards to the topic and issue covered. The publication is sold with the idea that the publisher is not required to render accounting, officially permitted, or otherwise, qualified services. If advice is necessary, legal or professional, a practiced individual in the profession should be ordered.

- From a Declaration of Principles which was accepted and approved equally by a Committee of the American Bar Association and a Committee of Publishers and Associations.

In no way is it legal to reproduce, duplicate, or transmit any part of this document in either electronic means or in printed format. Recording of this publication is strictly prohibited and any storage of this document is not allowed unless with written permission from the publisher. All rights reserved.

The information provided herein is stated to be truthful and consistent, in that any liability, in terms of inattention or otherwise, by any usage or abuse of any policies, processes, or directions contained within is the solitary and utter responsibility of the recipient reader. Under no circumstances will any legal responsibility or blame be held against the publisher for any reparation, damages, or monetary loss due to the information herein, either directly or indirectly.

Respective authors own all copyrights not held by the publisher.

The information herein is offered for informational purposes solely, and is universal as so. The presentation of the information is without contract or any type of guarantee assurance.

The trademarks that are used are without any consent, and the publication of the trademark is without permission or backing by the trademark owner. All trademarks and brands within this book are for clarifying purposes only and are the owned by the owners themselves, not affiliated with this document.

Chapter One: How to make Cauliflower Fried Rice

This recipe is ideal for those of you who are looking to cook some delicious and healthy food in a record time. This meal will supply you with the necessary fats and proteins that you will need and the macronutrients from this meal should offer you enough steam for the day. The best time to try this recipe is right after you finish your daily exercises.

List of Ingredients

50 Grams of bacon

200 Grams of cauliflower

80 Grams of onion

4 Tablespoons of water

200 Grams of frozen vegetables

30 Ml of liquid aminos

This recipe is easy to customize and you can use any type of vegetable and any type of meat. To begin with you will have to shred your cauliflower. I would advise you to use a grader with fairly large holes as you need to make sure that the cauliflower is properly crumbled.

It is now time to heat the pan. After you heat the pan you might want to add in the chopped onion. You will just want to saute it for a while. When your bacon is nice and crisp you know that it is time to add in the cauliflower. Finally you should give a really good stir for about five minutes.

After you add the bacon you might want to add just a couple of tablespoons of water just so that the food is nice and steamy. Let the cauliflower steam and add in any kind of vegetables that you may want. It is now time to add the frozen vegetables.

I will add about half a bag of frozen vegetables and I will give it a good stir. For the seasoning you can try to add fish sauce but my personal preference is liquid aminos. I hope that you will give this recipe a try and I am sure that you will love this recipe!

Chapter Two: How to make Raw Vegan Ground Meat

This raw vegan ground meat will add some delicious and chewy texture to any of your raw food recipes such as raw chili or even raw tacos. This type of recipe is really easy to prepare and as long as you have the ingredients at hand you can finish this recipe in only 25 minutes.

List of Ingredients

1 Clove of garlic

½ Cup of raw olives

4 Large button mushrooms

½ Teaspoon of cumin seed

2 Spoons of spice blend

2 Spoons of raw tomato ketchup

To begin with you will have to make the raw tomato ketchup. You may have to use a blender for this job but this is not mandatory. After I finish with the tomato ketchup I am going to throw in my cumin seed and half of a tea spoon of garlic powder. You can use any type of spice for this recipe, chili powder would also be great with this. I will also add in one clove of garlic.

After I finish adding all of the ingredients I am going to add three tablespoons of raw tomato ketchup. You can use any type of blender that you want and the key is to blend it for at least 30 seconds. You may not want to use it for more than 30 seconds because it will start to turn into a puree.

We will want this to be very grainy and meaty so we will just pulse it for a few times until everything gets blended together and forms a meaty texture. If you want to give your meat a special taste you may want to add some nuts and seeds but these are only optional. If you want your meat to have a stronger texture then you can mix the ingredients by hand.

This is the type of recipe that you can prepare early on in the morning. It is really easy to prepare and the only downside of this recipe lies in the ingredients because you will have to take your time to select this wide range of ingredients. Anyhow you can get this done in under 25 minutes and this is what I like the most about this recipe.

Chapter Three: How to make Delicious Paleo Donuts

I know that your first thought is that donuts are not healthy but if you use the proper ingredients you can create some absolutely delicious donuts that do not have any sort of extra calories, gluten and refined sugar.

List of Ingredients

¼ Teaspoon of baking soda

3 Tablespoons of pure maple syrup

¼ Teaspoon of almond extract

½ Teaspoon of vanilla extract

2 Tablespoons of coconut oil

1 Teaspoon of apple cider vinegar

2 Eggs

¼ Cup of unsweetened chocolate

2 Tablespoons of coconut oil

To begin with you will have to preheat the oven to 360 degrees Fahrenheit. Grease your six mold donut pan with coconut oil. After that, combine your dry ingredients into a medium bowl. In another bowl you should try to combine all the other ingredients and set up the egg whites.

It is now time to mix all the ingredients together and set them aside. Beat the egg whites until they are nice and soft. Gently fold the egg whites into the batter. Equally distribute the batter between the six donut molds and smooth out the top of each donut.

You should bake the donuts between 12 and 15 minutes until they turn into a light golden color. Allow the donuts to cool and remove them from the pan and let them chill in the refrigerator for about half an hour.

Place the glaze ingredients in a sauce pan and place the sauce pan into the skillet. Gently mix the ingredients until they are fully melted. Pour the melted chocolate into a bowl and gently dip each chilled donut into the chocolate.

Chapter Four: How to make Sweet Potato Bacon Cakes

If you are looking for a quick and delicious snack then you should definitely learn how to make some sweet potato bacon cakes. These cakes will sweeten out your day and they won't add those extra calories that we all hate. This is the ideal snack to serve early on in the morning.

List of Ingredients

1 Teaspoon of cinnamon

2 Teaspoons of baking powder

500 Grams of sweet potato

3 Cups of flower

½ Teaspoon of baking soda

2 Cups of sugar

1 Cup of butter

1 Teaspoon of vanilla extract

2 Eggs

To begin with you will have to peel your sweet potatoes and then simply place them in a hot pan and cook them. It is now time to use a bowl and add three cups of flour and two cups of baking powder. You will also have to add one teaspoon of cinnamon and half a teaspoon of baking soda and ¼ teaspoon of salt.

It is now time to thoroughly mix all of the ingredients. In another bowl you should add two cups of sugar and one cup of butter. And mix them up. It is now time to add 1 teaspoon of vanilla extract and mix the ingredients really well.

After you mix all the ingredients you should add two eggs and continue to mix for a few minutes. After you are done with mixing you can use another bowl to mash all of the potatoes. You need to get them mashed really well and then add 2 cups of sweet potatoes to the mixture and mix it until it is nice and smooth.

Finally, you need to transfer the mix to your baking pan and bake at 350 degrees for 15 minutes. In the end you should have your fast, delicious and easy to prepare sweet potato cake. I really hope that you will enjoy this recipe as this is one of my all-time favorites.

Chapter Five: How to make Chicken Sushi

This chicken sushi is really easy to make and this type of food would be ideal to serve during the afternoon after you finish your exercises. This meal is extremely rich in lean protein and this is why I would highly recommend it after an exhausting session at the gym.

List of Ingredients

50 Ml of sesame seed oil

200 Grams of chicken

30 Ml of sweet teriyaki sauce

1 Sheet of nori

50 Ml of vinegar

50 Grams of sliced cucumber

100 Grams of boiled rice

50 Grans if sesame seeds

- In order to fry the chicken you need to mix it with some hot sesame oil. You will want your chicken to be cooked but not over cooked because if you overcook the chicken it will be very dry. Finally you need to flip the chicken and add some teriyaki sauce.

- It is now time to set the chicken aside and start rolling a bamboo rolling mat. You will have to place a sheet of nori on top of the bamboo mat. You will now take the sushi rice and you will spread it out evenly over your nori sheet. Flip the rice sheet over and place two pieces of chicken along with some sliced cucumber.

- Finally, you will have to roll the bamboo sheet and compress it. In the end you will have to cut the sushi roles in thin pieces. The ideal width should be of about 1 inch. Anyway it is now time to get the sushi and add it on your plate.

- If you want to give your sushi roles a really special taste you can try to add just a little bit of ginger. You should drizzle some teriyaki sauce over the sushi roles and this will give your sushi roles a really glossy and sweet honey like aspect. In the end you can sprinkle some freshly roasted sesame seeds on top of the sushi roles.

Chapter Six: The Frugal Breakfast of Your Dreams

This recipe revolves around one thing – budget. If you want to have something healthy but you are on a low budget than you should definitely learn how to use this recipe. I have used this recipe when I was in college and I still use it when I am extremely busy early on in the morning. This breakfast should last you for at least three days and this is the most positive aspect of this recipe.

List of Ingredients

250 Grams of hash browns

200 Grams of bacon

250 Grams of brie

10 Eggs

30 Grams of butter

The first thing that you need to do is to cook your bacon. While your bacon is cooking you can prepare your eggs inside of your muffin pan. You need to stir your eggs inside of the muffin hole. When the bacon is done cooking move it to the side and let it to cool down.

I would recommend cooking your eggs in your bacon grease because they will taste better and they will be crispier as well. You should make sure to cut your bacon into really small pieces. It is now time to sprinkle a little bit of bacon onto the eggs that you have in your muffin holes.

The last thing that you are going to add is your brie cheese. You should make sure to shred your brie cheese before adding it to the mix. You will need to mix everything really well because if you do not mix the ingredients everything will go out of proportion and it won't taste as good. You will then have to place the muffin holes inside the oven and bake them at 350 degrees for about 16 minutes.

When you get the muffin holes out of the oven you are done. You may want to use a sandwich bag in order to preserve this food. This meal will last you for at least three days and you will not have to prepare the breakfast food every morning. It is natural to assume that you can serve this meal with some vegetables and this is quite an important aspect. I like to serve this food with some chili and tomato.

Chapter Seven: How to Make Easy Chicken Curry

If you are looking to lose a lot of weight fast you should definitely try out this recipe. Chicken meat has a low number of calories and if you are looking to lose a lot of weight fast this recipe is ideal for you. I have managed to lose 2 pounds/week and this recipe has helped me quite a lot.

List of Ingredients

50 Grams of onion

70 Grams of cucumber

250 Grams of chicken

2 Cloves of garlic

20 Grams of curry spice

50 Grams of tomatoes

100 Grams of fat free yogurt

150 Grams of mushrooms

First of all you will have to chop all of your ingredients into similar sized pieces. After you are done with chopping the ingredients you should place a pan on a low heat. Lightly mist the pan with some low calorie cooking spray or olive oil.

After the pan has reached the boiling point you should add the onion and gently mix it for one minute. After that you should add the cucumber and the chicken. Make sure to mix it really well before you finally add the garlic.

It is now time to add the tomatoes and curry spice. Make sure to stir fry all the ingredients for three minutes. If you notice that the vegetables start to stick to the pan you should try to add a splash of water. Towards the end of the cooking process you can add the mushrooms and keep on mixing the ingredients until the mushrooms are nice and brown.

If you notice that the meat starts to form a yellow brown color than you should know that it is time to lift the pan from the heat and add some chopped tomatoes and stock. Make sure to simmer for 30 minutes before finally lifting the pan. In the end you can two spoons of fat free yogurt.

Chapter Eight: How to Make Chili con Carne

All of us love to eat tasty food but the problem with tasty food lies in the number of calories. This recipe is very low in calories and it is really tasty. If you want to maintain your weight and if you love spicy food then you are definitely going to enjoy this recipe. This food is like a one pot wonder as it is really easy to prepare and it is packed with flavor.

List of Ingredients

50 Grams of onion

50 Grams of garlic

500 Grams of beef

80 Grams of chili

50 Grams of hot pepper

120 Grams of tomato

80 Ml of stock

250 Grams of kidney beans

To begin with you should fry the onion and garlic until they turn golden yellow. After you are done with the onion and garlic you should add the beef and cook for a few minutes on high heat. When your beef is browned you should add your chili and spices and turn down the heat.

It is now time to add the peppers, tomatoes and stock. After you add these make sure to simmer gently for 15 minutes until the sauce is reduced. Finally, add the kidney beans for 5 minutes before the end just to make sure that they are warmed through. In the end you can top it with a swirl of fat free fromage frais and sprinkle it with chopped herbs and paprika. You can serve this food on a large jacket potato with lots of rice.

Chapter Nine: How to Make Caribbean Stew

I am a big fan of food from the Caribbean as the flavor and color of this food is absolutely outstanding. This Caribbean stew is absolutely delicious and I would highly recommend it if you want to eat something truly tasty. This stew is very easy to make and it is quite low in terms of calories.

List of Ingredients

300 Grams of beef

2 Garlic cloves

60 Grams of chili

40 Grams of onion

150 Ml of beef stock

150 Grams of sweet potato

½ Teaspoon of sweetener

50 Ml of red wine

Start by removing all the fat off the beef. After you are done with the beef you should peel and prepare the vegetables. It would be great if you can cut them into evenly sized pieces. The meat and vegetables should be cut into similar sized pieces.

If you cut the meat and the beef in similar sized pieces everything will cook evenly. It is now time to spray the casserole dish with low calorie cooking spray and drop in the beef over a medium to high heat. When the meat turns brown you should add the rest of the vegetables.

After you give it a good mix for a few minutes you should add some spices. Season and cook on a low heat for about 90 minutes. If you notice that the beef is soft and tender than you should turn down the heat and remove the pan.

It is wise to choose slow cooking for this recipe because the meat will tenderize and it would be a lot tastier because the meat flavor will blend in with the rest of the ingredients. You can serve this recipe as it is or with a big bowl of boiled rice.

Best Practices & Common Dieting Mistakes

In this chapter you are going to learn some tricks that will help you to lose weight as fast as possible. I know that a lot of you people think that dieting is tough but you can view it in a different way. If you view dieting as a game with its own set of rules you will realize that you can lose weight much faster.

Do's

Count Your Calories

It is extremely important to count your calories every day. If you count your calories with a special app you will know what type of foods will make you fat and white type of foods will help you to lose weight.

Eat More Foods with Natural Sugar

There are a plethora of foods that come in with natural sugars and these foods are all created by nature. Natural sugar or fructose is packed with vitamins and nutrients that will help you to maintain your weight and natural sugars are absorbed more slowly, unlike man-made sugars.

Motivation is Key

This is the most important aspect and if you are strongly focused on the main reason that motivates you to lose weight you will be successful.

Don'ts

Select a weak Reason to Lose Weight

If you want to stay motivated through your weight loss journey you should select a very strong reason that motivates you to lose weight.

Eat out in Town

One of the main reasons for failed diets is laziness. People are simply bored of making their own food and they choose to eat out in town.

Think that it Might Happen Over Night

Losing weight is all about goal setting. If you have a really strong goal then you should divide that goal into daily micro goals.

What's next?

Tips & Tricks for Effortless Cooking

I've used to work as a professional chef for years and I can tell you that there are a lot of tips and tricks that you can use in order to cook your food fast. I know that many people ignore the overall quality of their kitchen equipment and this is a big mistake.

If you want to cook fast you should definitely invest in a high quality set of knives. A good knife will cost between 50$ and 200$. I would advise you to choose a Japanese or German knife company because they manufacture remarkable knives.

I know that the average person does not afford to buy a 150$ knife but the truth is that you will save a lot of time if you have the proper tools and you can use that time for other purposes. Moreover cooking will become truly effortless. Think about the time that you can save when deboning a fish or a chicken. With a good knife you can save at least 40 minutes during this process.

If you want to practice effortless cooking you should form the habit of cooking simple and nutritious recipes. This is why I have shared some very simple recipes with you. Dieting is all about cooking your own nutritious and natural food and the concept of easy cooking is relatively new in the world of dieting.

When it comes to effortless cooking you need to find simple recipes and you need to be able to invest more money in your kitchen. If you still have a rudimentary kitchen it is not that easy to cook simple and delicious food and you will definitely have to make a change.

The future of cooking will revolve around simplicity and time. The time factor will be extremely important because let's face it – cooking takes a lot of time and preparing healthy food takes even more. We are still far from the day when robots will take over our kitchens and we will have to fend for ourselves.

The most important thing that you can do in order to practice effortless cooking is to learn at least 10 healthy and easy ways to prepare food. If you learn these recipes in one month and if you practice them every day you will manage to cook healthy food in a few minutes. Practice makes perfect and nowhere in the world is this statement more important than in the world of cooking.

All in all, if you want to stay in shape and if you want to practice effortless cooking you should think about allocating more resources for your kitchen. Imagine that you make this investment for your health and think about the long time consequences of your action. You should also try to keep in mind that everything that is truly worth doing is worth doing poor at the very beginning.

Conclusion

I hope that this book has brought a fresh perspective in your overall vision of effortless cooking. Keep in mind that just like anything else in the world, cooking and dieting take time to perfect. Take your time and learn how to cook some healthy food and you will immediately rip the benefits and you will also learn a skill that will be appreciated by everyone around you.

If you take the time to discipline yourself in order to lose weight and if you take the time to learn new recipes you will feel better about yourself. You will notice this positive wave of energy that will radiate around you and everyone will start to love you and appreciate you for your effort.

I have a very strong opinion about the type of food that my family should enjoy. My ideal version of a meal would be of something that is healthy, easy to prepare and affordable. Healthy food should not burn a hole in your pocket and it should not take more than a few minutes to prepare. After all, you could use the rest of your time for things that are far more important.

If you feel as if the food that you prepare is turning your life into a nightmare than you should try to solve this problem. Cooking takes time and we spend a lot of time in our kitchen. In order to lead a successful life we need to take control of our life and we need to control each and every aspect of it.

If you start to control your cooking and if you try to improve your skills you will save a lot of time and you will learn how to prepare delicious foods in no time. Just like in any other aspect of our life, time is essential and spending too much time on a particular task and you will start to develop a negative mindset. This negative mindset may affect your opinion about a thing that can turn out to be your next big passion.

I have discovered that many successful people had a lot of moments when they were confused and lost and they began to hate their job. Your duty is to stay smart and figure out why you cannot keep your diet or why you cannot easily cook simple and delicious food. If you begin to work on this problem right now you will start to lose weight and you will also develop a skill that will stay with you for the rest of your life.

In the end, nobody was born perfect and nobody was born to be a perfect chef and for everything in this world there was a beginning. Now is the best time for you to begin to learn how to master the art of cooking. I hope that this book has helped you to develop a vision of healthy eating as this is the vision that has helped me to lose my extra pounds and now I can enjoy my version of an ideal life.

Thank you again for downloading this book!

I hope this book was able to help you make delicious bulletproof recipes that you will make again and again...while being frugal and fast and easy.

The next step is to apply the knowledge learned in this book. Keep a positive outlook have fun discovering how the bulletproof diet can help you to reclaim your focus and energy.

Before you go, I'd like to say thank you for purchasing my book.

I know you could have picked so many other books to read on the bulletproof diet, but you took a chance on me.

So A Big thanks for downloading this book and reading it all the way to completion.

Now I would like to ask a _small_ favor.

Could you please take a minute or two to leave a review for this book on Amazon?

The feedback will help me continue to publish more kindle books that will help people to get better results in their lives.

And if you found it helpful in anyway then please let me know :-)

Thank you and good luck!

Preview of my New Book

Yoga For Beginners: The Ultimate Yoga Guide for Newbies: How To Relieve Stress, Lose Weight, and find Inner Peace

This book contains proven steps and strategies on how to practice yoga. You will learn how to achieve inner peace, while living a stress free life and perhaps begin to lose weight with the continuing practice of yoga.

In this book we will offer an explanation of the Yoga technique. By reading this book you will be able to learn how to practice the basics of the technique in order to get balance back to your body and mind. By following these simple steps you could possibly find a new you. You don`t need any money, a lot of time or effort, you just have to start to love and practice Yoga.

Click here to get your copy.

More Books by Michele Gilbert

Below you'll find some of my other books that are popular on Amazon and Kindle Simply click on the links below to check them out.

Practicing Mindfulness: Living in the moment through Meditation: Everyday Habits and Rituals to help you achieve inner peace

Sleep Tight: Overcome Insomnia and Sleep Disorders for a better more restful sleep!

Stop Back Pain Now!: Back Pain Remedies and Treatments so you can live a pain free life!

The Arthritis Pain Cure: How to find Arthritis Pain Relief and live a happy pain free life!

The Headache Pain Cure: How to find Headache Pain Relief and live a happy Pain Free Life!

Stop Panic Attacks and Anxiety Disorders without Drugs Now!: Overcome Panic, Stress and Anxiety and live a happy pain free life!

The Breakup Recovery Guide: Advice for Surviving Heartbreak, Letting Go and Thriving in an exciting new life!

The Friendship Guide to Finding Friends Forever: How to Find, Make and Keep Quality Friendships After your Breakup

The Credit Fix: Leave behind credit card debt and poor credit scores and get your life back!

www.ingramcontent.com/pod-product-compliance
Lightning Source LLC
Chambersburg PA
CBHW050911290526
45792CB00002B/777